Vibrant

Developing and Perfecting Yourself

(Book Two)

Dr. Josefina Monasterio

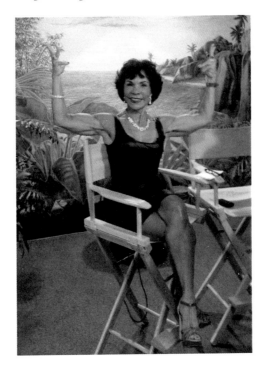

What Others Have to Say

The rest of your life is in your hands, no one else's. I share what others are saying to encourage you. You can change your life to whatever you want it to be.

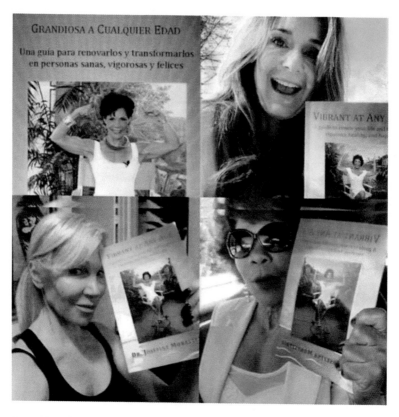

Josefina, I am a Registered Nurse as well as a fitness instructor who has been working out for 32 years. I just want you to know what an inspiration you are. I will be buying your book and sharing it. You look amazing and give hope to others who feel like getting in shape is impossible. So many people complain they can't diet and lose weight, but eating clean is a lifestyle. Thank you for inspiring me. K.

Good morning Josefina, I loved the whole book! So much of it resonated with me. I woke up this morning thinking about something that was disturbing me. So I referred to that page in your book and I released it! I'm now relaxing in silence and starting my day. Thank you again, and have a fabulous day. POW!

Josefina Monasterio, my mom took my copy and is reading it now! I told her that I ordered a signed copy for her but she won't let go of my copy. She says, "That Josefina is one more smart woman!" Hopefully she will finish it today so I can read it. J.S.

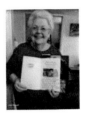

I have always heard the saying, *Age is just a number*, until I followed you, after which I'm darn sure that it's just a useless number.

I came across your profile during a business seminar. The speaker quoted you regarding his life experience. It's never too late to start believing in your will power. Well done darling.

Thank you Dr. Josefina. I enjoyed watching your video, and I'm ready to improve how I live. One thing I got from you that I always hold onto is, *Never give up!* C.B

I bought your book yesterday on Amazon. I am halfway through. While working cutting hair I recommend it to my clients. Your book reads genuine, heartfelt, and it is motivational. What a great foundation for people of all ages. M.D.

I just started following you on Facebook - saw your story. I am in awe of you, your discipline, and dedication to fitness. I'm 52 and want to get in the best shape of my life. I'm going to buy your book. You are my inspiration and a role model to all women! Thank you. D.M.

I have bought your book. I am on an incredible journey of health and personal development. The only way is forward and at 72 I am not looking back. Enjoy your day and best wishes from lovely Australia. S.G.

I believe in you Josefina. I love the way you live life. You have helped us all. P.S.

I just heard about you this morning. You are one of the more interesting people I've seen in a long time. You have inspired me to get back into body building in my 30s. C.

Got the book and am reading it. Insightful and well-written. I need motivation. M.G.

So glad I found your website. My friends take the senior discount, but it felt wrong when I took it, like something inside me was breaking. Now, after seeing you on YouTube, I am stoked to re-build my lost muscle mass and return to my "young thinking, acting, and being." B.N.

Girl, I just want to tell you how you have been pushing me! I saw a video about who you are, how old you are, and what you do. I wake up now looking forward to my workouts. And during my walks with my neighbor I'm motivating her now.

Hi Josefina, I just finished your first book and it is so inspirational. I love the way you live your life and am going to apply your principles to mine. Your book is bringing about a powerful paradigm shift. It's on now! P.G.

Our priorities, our lives, and our idols change as time passes. My priority now is health and family. And my idol is Dr. Josefina Monasterio.

You have clearly defied the laws of aging—or reversed them! J.F.

This is so good. You have motivated me to fitness. I have been fit before. I will do so again. Thanks. A.W.

ISBN-13: 978-1721192441

Vibrant at Any Age series

Book One: *Vibrant at Any Age: A guide to renew your life and become vigorous, healthy, and happy* (English and Spanish editions)

Book Two: *Vibrant Learning: Developing and Perfecting Yourself* (English and Spanish editions)

Book Three: *Vibrant Relationships for Healthy and Powerful Living*

You can reach Dr. Josefina at DrJosefinaMonasterio@gmail.com

Website: www.DrJosefina.com
Facebook: www.facebook.com/drjosefina
Twitter: www.twitter.com/drjosefina
YouTube: www.youtube.com/drjosefina
LinkedIn: www.linkedin.com/in/dr-josefina-monasterio-a69baa16/
Instagram: www.instagram.com/drjosefinamonasterio/

To be vibrant you must cultivate your whole being: physical, emotional, mental, and spiritual. There are laws that govern your physical fitness, mental health, and spiritual maturity. Your efforts to comply with these laws determine your well being.

Contents

Introduction: Keep Learning

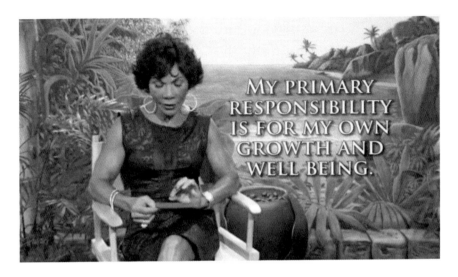

MY PRIMARY RESPONSIBILITY IS FOR MY OWN GROWTH AND WELL BEING.

Intellectual growth should commence at birth and cease
only at death. (Albert Einstein)

This is the second book in the series, *Vibrant at Any Age*. My purpose is to share the nuts and bolts of building a better you and inspire a passion for learning. But it's up to you to **keep learning**. Don't worry, as Leonardo da Vinci said, "Learning never exhausts the mind" (although sometimes mine does get weary).

Why it is so powerful to keep learning?

You are responsible for your growth and well-being. You have a physical body with a mind and a spirit seated on it. Exercising your body, developing your mind, and growing in spirit keeps you up to date, feeling a part of society, and not an old person huddled in a corner. It breaks the stereotype that an old dog can't learn new tricks. Don't you believe it. It is totally false. Bow wow!

Learning and the aging process

It is good for your brain to keep learning. You've no doubt heard that as you grow older that the connections in the brain became fixed (arthritis comes to mind), and then it's just a matter of time until you really start losing brain cells. A recipe for going downhill for sure. How discouraging. But like many things we once believed, I'm glad to tell you it's not so.

We're learning a lot about nerve cell development as people age. Crystallized and fluid intelligence show that in youth we are better at memorizing information. And as we grow older we become better at evaluating information and putting it into practice. Neurogenesis or brain plasticity means that the brain changes throughout life by forming new connections among brain cells, which changes how we do things.

The brain never stops changing. It continues to grow no matter how old you are. If your mental capacity is decreasing, there are physical changes in the brain that are causing it. Fortunately, you can avoid and even reverse this problem with physical and mental training exercises for the brain. The key is to challenge the brain, to do novel and stimulating tasks that do not rely on established ways of doing things. Think new, do new, be new.

Some other benefits of learning

If you choose to stay in the workforce you need to be up to date on our rapidly changing technology. Education becomes imperative. Even in retirement, this era of technology requires learning new things to enrich your life and leisure activities. Many older adults are attending college classes to enhance their lives. That's awesome!

Another benefit to keep on learning is that you develop a social network that allows you to share your time, knowledge, and have fun activities. It adds meaning to what you do every day. We need to be with other people because we are social beings.

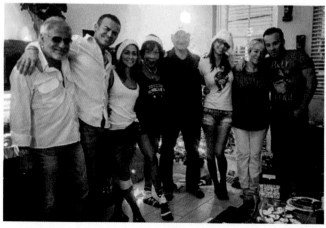

Seek to include in your social network people younger than yourself. A different generation keeps you up to date with what's trending, the pulse of what's happening in society that you wouldn't know about otherwise.

Interacting with people of different backgrounds, different genders, and different races broadens your view of the world. The diversity enriches your life and keeps you feeling happy, healthy, and terrific—vibrant! And at the same time you contribute to others with your life experience. It's a win-win, wouldn't you say?

So what's the point to keep learning? Learning is exercise for the brain. It makes you more social. You live your life as an exclamation point!!!!!

POW!

Keep Learning about Nutrition

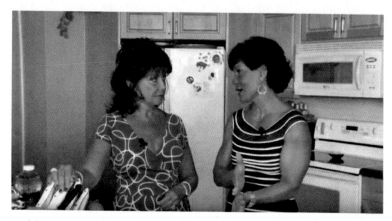

Taking care of yourself means learning about nutrition. It takes effort and commitment but it is well worth it. You don't have to be a nutritionist; you just need to find out what works for you. It is a lifelong endeavor because our nutritional needs change as the years pass.

I stay away from processed foods. I would not even call them food because real food keeps us healthy and does not make us sick. Genuine food is the source of our energy, which enables us to achieve our daily purpose. Processed foods are extremely dangerous to our health. They lack nutritional value. Worse, they are loaded with artificial coloring, chemicals, sugar, and high levels of sodium that preserves them for ages. These things cause many diseases, such as cancer, diabetes, loss of bone density—and a lot more. No wonder people die miserably.

As a rule I eat foods that are natural and fresh. I seldom eat out. I'd rather prepare my meals to be sure that what I eat is exactly what my body needs. But I do eat out after my competitions. I treat myself to chicken quesadilla, chips, salsa. For a drink I have a mojito; I ask it to be made with real rum and not a chemicalized drink mix. For desert I have flan or dulce de leche. This is the only time I eat out.

My grocery shopping is mostly the same. It takes me less than a half-hour because I know exactly where to go. I walk through the aisles only when I need products for the house. But when starting out with a new way to eat, you must find where the things you want are kept. After that it's easy to do your food shopping.

I prefer my veggies to be organic. You can taste the difference; it's humongous. I like broccoli, cauliflower, green beans, spinach, avocado, onions, garlic, and sweet potatoes. I have the same approach when it comes to getting my proteins, like meat. The best protein biologically speaking is eggs. I find these foods in my local super market; I don't make a special trip to get my groceries.

People often ask me to share with them what I eat. I am happy to tell you, but I have learned what works for me may not work for you. It can serve only as a guide and a motivation to eat healthy. It's why you need to be careful and not blindly copy what I or anyone else does.

I'll tell you how I discovered the nutritional formula that works for me. But I started wrong and had to learn the hard way (not uncommon, is it?). It began with my bodybuilding career. I saw most bodybuilders eating rice and I thought, *That's what I need, it has to be good for me.*

Wrong! Wrong! Wrong! One-half hour after I ate my meal with rice I was hungry again; and it happened over and over. I finally learned that rice raises my blood sugar a few minutes after eating. POW! I would come crashing down and be hungry again.

After trying different carbohydrates, I discovered that what works best for me is sweet potatoes. It keeps my blood sugar stable for about 2½ hours and then I eat something. Another food that works great for me is chicken. These two foods are part of my daily meals, along with broccoli, cauliflower, onions, and other veggies.

For breakfast what works for me is oatmeal, the old fashion kind. I rarely eat processed food. I stay as close to nature as I can to maintain a healthy body and mind. For snacks I am a fruit lover: bananas, mangos peaches, nectarines, pineapples and blueberries are among my favorites.

I like nuts. But I'm careful not to eat too many, usually as snacks. I don't like to consume oils in liquid form (that's just me), so nuts are a delicious way to "eat" my oils. And being real food there is less opportunity of man's involvement and so it's better for me. Brazil nuts are a powerhouse of nutrients. Cashews are part of my ritual when I am competing. I also eat them as an energy snack; sometimes I add honey or a quality marmalade; it's divine.

You cannot afford to be lazy about discovering the blueprint of your nutritional plan. I recommend to my clients that they keep a log to discover what works for them. Unfortunately, most people won't take the time. I see their faces unhappy and eyes rolling when I asked them to diary what they eat. Keep a log for three days and record how you feel. How hard can that be?

Sometimes we don't want to face reality. That way it's easy to blame your genetics: "Oh well, it is what it is." I say stop it! Take responsibility; take charge of the things you have control over. By becoming accountable for the smalls things, you are creating the foundation for the big ones: a healthy, youthful, and ageless life.

Preparing your own food

Now that we learned what to eat, it makes sense that preparing your own food ensures you'll eat exactly what you want, what you should, and what you need. Eating out is a fun way to be with others, but it's a challenge to keep it healthy. But if you normally eat what you should, then eating the things that are bad for you once in a while won't be a problem.

I prepare most of my food at home. Here are some videos about how I do it.

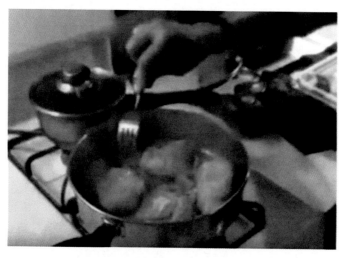

Easy healthy nutritious meals
(http://bit.ly/MealsDrJ)

Keep Learning about Sleep

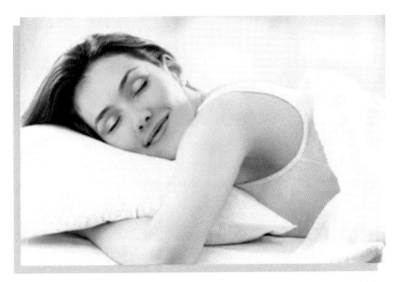

Resting is as important as being active. The body builds and repairs itself when we sleep. The brain deletes all the junk accumulated during the day. It is the time for the production of human growth hormone and the rejuvenation of muscles. The release of melatonin occurs right before you drift off to dreamland. However, this natural hormone does far more than simply whisk you away to la-la land with a flush of feel good emotions. Melatonin has numerous health benefits. It infuses the immune system with a powerful flush of antioxidants that fight free radical damage, cancer, inflammation, and brain decline.

How you approach sleep determines how effective its benefits are. As I do at the beginning of my day, I approach my night rest with a ritual that prepares me for sleep. Following these steps each evening makes it more likely that I will sleep well through the night. I do these activities with reverence, grateful that I have had one more day to do good and be my best.

This is my ritual:

- I clean my face. I never go to sleep with my face covered with makeup. The skin needs to breathe to be rejuvenated and restored.
- I avoid watching TV or using the computer, smart phone, or tablet an hour or so before going to bed. If I do watch

something, I make sure it does not disturb my mind; only things that are lovely and gracious.

- I sleep in complete darkness—or as close to it as possible. Even the tiniest glow from a clock can disturb your sleep. So cover it at night or get rid of it.

- I keep the temperature in my bedroom below 70 degrees F. Many people keep their homes too warm, particularly upstairs bedrooms. Studies show that the optimal room temperature for sleep is 60-68 degrees.

- After I take care of my physical body, I get into a state of calm: relaxed body, quiet mind, and grateful spirit. I thank God for the blessings, successes, and my strength during the day. I call it the *Value of the Day*.

Remember your mom saying, "Get your beauty sleep?" She was right. Just remember how you feel and look when you have a lousy, sleepless night. I rest my case. Learn the good that a tiptop night of sleep does to your body, mind, and spirit.

Keep Learning about Fitness

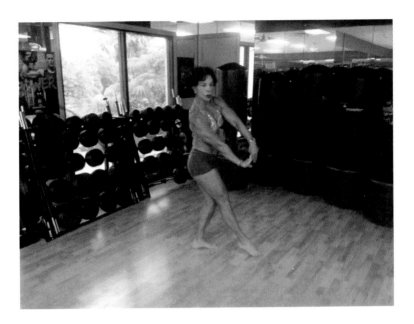

Working out in the gym

If you want to achieve results in the gym, be clear in your purpose so you approach your gym time with respect—almost reverence. It is not a time to socialize and chitchat. It won't give you the results you want. The gym is where you take care of your health—and your health is sacred.

I find it pathetic and insulting when I watch personal trainers talk with their clients about matters that have nothing to do with their health and well-being; they should be correcting the form of the person doing the exercises. When you hire a personal trainer be sure it is to train your muscles and transform your body. Why waste your time and money if that's not your attitude?

One of my clients wanted to develop discipline and commitment to her fitness. Well, almost every week she would tell me her personal trainer couldn't make it because of some personal issue. That went on for about six months. And that wasn't all. In one of our sessions I brought it to her attention that her trainer was failing her; instead of reinforcing good habits she was doing the opposite. Grrr! So I suggested she fire her trainer. And she did!

Your trainer, your coach, and the people around you must be aligned with your goals and purposes if you are going to be successful.

When you are shopping for a gym here are some things to keep in mind.

- Look for free weights and benches with different sets of dumbbells.
- There should be exercise machines and cable setups that allow you to work all parts of your body.
- Is there an area where you can do your cardiovascular training: treadmills, exercise bikes, steppers, aerobic classes—whatever you need to get your heart going and take care of your body?
- Make sure you like the atmosphere, the feng shui of the gym and the building. You want to feel like it's your second home.
- Check other amenities important to you, such as a swimming pool, massage, tennis, volleyball, and so on.

If you are self-directed, you can set up a home gym. But you have to be dead serious about spending all that money so you can have a place to hang your dirty clothes. I prefer to go to the gym. Luckily, in my town we have an incredibly complete gym. It's perfect for my needs.

What should you wear?

Dress for the gym with clothes that fit your body and make you feel great! Be mindful of looking your best each time you go to do your work out. Why? Because it's a big motivator. You feel good about yourself; you feel you are making progress. You are dressing for that special occasion, your journey of developing and perfecting.

Have a mental picture of your goal. It can be someone you admire and respect; or it can be your own picture, a time when you were in the best shape and looking good.

Get quality shoes, gloves, straps and belts. But don't go crazy. Before you go shopping, while working out in the gym, decide what you need—and then shop. Why waste your time and money!

If you have long hair, make sure it's out of the way. You should be focused on the task in front of you, not dealing with your hair. Avoid distractions of any kind because they take your energy. My gym energy is for training my muscles. It's crucial to have a mind-muscle connection (that means no mind distractions) to achieve the results you want.

Workout videos

Here are videos of how I work out different parts of my body.

Abdominals Core Muscles (http://bit.ly/Abdominals-DrJ)	Back workout (http://bit.ly/Back-DrJ)
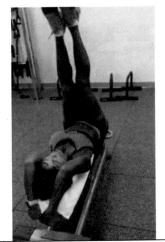	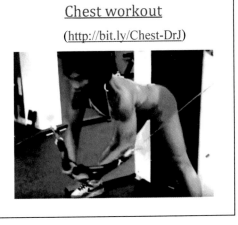
Shoulders workout (http://bit.ly/Shoulders-DrJ)	Chest workout (http://bit.ly/Chest-DrJ)
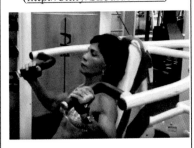	

Legs workout
(http://bit.ly/Legs-DrJ)

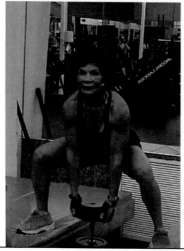

Workout for beginners
(http://bit.ly/BeginnersDrJ)

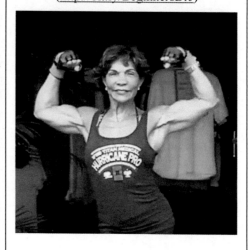

Yoga
(http://bit.ly/YogaDrJ)

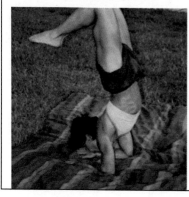

RESERVED FOR YOU

Be inspired as you watch them. Find what works for you.

Keep Looking your Best

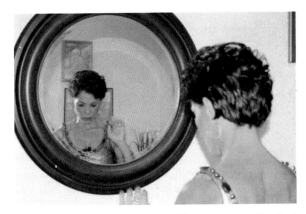

You feel wonderful about yourself when you look the best you can. You radiate feelable confidence and energy. Friends, family, and acquaintances respond; they want to be near you. You glow with the poise of a person who knows where he or she is going. I learned this from my friend Rosie.

Years ago I took no care of how I looked when I went about my errands. It didn't matter how others saw me. One day Rosie lovingly said, "Josefina, you are well known in the community, you have a TV show, you are a life coach, you need to change how you look. POW! That was a whack on the side of the head.

From that moment on, whenever I go out, no matter the reason or how short the errand, I go looking my best, even to the gym.

People go out of their way to help me to find what I need. I confess it's a pain sometimes. I want to be left alone, not having someone ask me every minute, *Am I finding everything?* Trust me, I would let them know; I'm not bashful as you may have noticed. It's at times like these when I notice that less attractive people receive less attention.

As you age it becomes more important to look and feel good to break stereotypes about aging. Looking your best improves how you feel about yourself. You thereby earn self-respect and also gain the respect of others. Self-respect is how you see yourself, and it affects how others see you. What an incredible effect it has knowing who you are and liking what you see. People are drawn to confident people. It makes them happy when they find it in you, and they enjoy being with you.

There are several ways to gain the confidence that comes from self-respect. The one we're discussing is showing yourself attractively. First because it makes you feel good, and then because you have only one chance to make a first impression—that's why it's call a *first* impression.

What's the biggest turnoff when first meeting a person? Bad hygiene. It means many things, such as bad breath, ill-fitting clothes, unkempt hair. You are in control; you can eliminate *turn-off* and replace it with *turn-on* by presenting the best possible version of yourself.

Being physically attractive is only the beginning of expanding your social network. It extends to strong character, which comes from the choices you have made and the values you have acquired. It results in attributes like kindness, generosity, empathy, modesty, and poise. People will be drawn to you and you will meet engaging people. So will your connections with others increase and open new and exciting avenues in your life. You will enrich their lives and they will enhance yours.

Take time to enjoy the company of those already in your circle of acquaintances and friends. You also want to enlarge the circle until you feel satisfied. But first you need to meet people. You do this by networking. We're social beings; that's how we are made. That means it's important that people enjoy your company. People like people who show themselves friendly. People care about those who care about them. It's simple: be genuinely interested in others. It's a form of love.

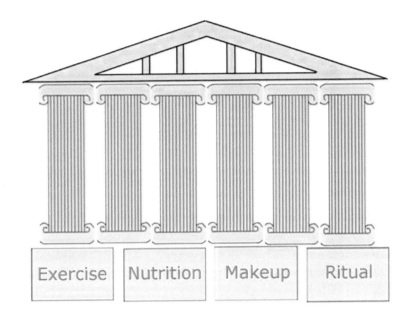

Exercise | Nutrition | Makeup | Ritual

Exercise

My first beauty tip is to exercise every day for vitality, balance, and beautiful skin. I have been involved in sports all my life, and one change I noticed very early was the difference of my skin after physical activity. Your skin looks radiant, younger, and healthy. That's a great incentive to start or continue exercising.

Nutrition

My second tip—you probably guessed it—is nutrition. You have no doubt heard that beauty comes from within. That's the truth—as within, so without. Nutrition is monumental in how healthy you look and feel.

As you know by now, I do not eat processed foods. I stay as close to nature as I can, making my own meals, and I seldom eat out. The only canned foods I purchase to make cooking easier are tomatoes or a nice salsa with only salt added.

These are foods that make for a healthy skin:

- Fruit—Eat fruits that are high in carotenoids. You will know them by their colors: red, orange, and yellow. You'll end up with a glow and will look healthier than having a tan.
- Nuts—Because of their dense nutritional value, nuts are part of any beauty regimen. It's also the antioxidant activity that is so beneficial, especially almonds. It deals with those pesky free radicals that make your skin look old (Ugh!). Vitamin E in nuts helps your skin hold in its moisture. Walnuts are also good for your skin.
- Red and Green Vegetables—Orange and red vegetables have plenty of beta-carotene. Your body makes it into vitamin A, which prevents cell damage and premature aging. Spinach and other green, leafy foods also provide lots of vitamin A.
- Citrus Fruits—Your skin needs collagen for its structure. It is the vitamin C in citrus that helps produce it. If you don't have enough it leads to sagging skin. But it's never too late to begin because vitamin C helps tighten skin at any age. I often use lemon in my tea and cooking to add vitamin C.
- Drink high quality water to keep your skin moist. I don't follow a protocol of how many glasses I should drink in a day. I listen to my body; when I am thirsty I drink. The exception is when I am working out; then I drink water after almost every set. It's crucial to keep your muscles hydrated.
- Stay away from drugs and alcohol. They'll do a number on your skin. Same with processed foods and trans fat.

Choosing the best quality food makes a huge difference. When it comes to nutrition it's all about eating foods in their natural state as much as you can. God made food, not man!

Makeup

Another one of my beauty tips is that I never go to bed with makeup on my face. It is a big factor that causes premature aging. I learned this from my mother. I was fascinated as a child watching her nightly ritual of cleaning her face.

I would hear conversations between my mom and friends and relatives discussing the latest beauty products. But it's from my grandmother that I drew wisdom. In particular, coconut oil. POW! She used it on her hair and skin. Her skin was beautifully smooth and silky. And she had few white hairs, if any! As a young woman I tried so many products. You name it and I tried it. I finally realized that the best product, at least for me, is coconut oil moisturizer. My grandma was right! Now I use coconut oil as a cleanser, moisturizer, and it is the oil you see on my skin when I compete.

I learned about coconut oil from watching my grandmother make it. She would pick up a fallen coconut, break it open, extract the meat, grind it, and then squeeze out the milk. Then she would cook it until the oil separated. The result was *pure* coconut oil, the real deal!

Ritual

Ok, now we need to add another pillar to beauty—ritual. Make sure to regularly get your beauty sleep and minimize stress daily in your life by following the meditation I share later in this book.

In summary, your beauty program should consist of:
- daily exercise
- natural foods
- coconut oil as makeup
- sleep
- meditation

From this blue print you will create an awesome program, one that works for you. My philosophy, keep it simple!

A reminder: beauty comes from the inside

I didn't feel beautiful when I was pregnant. I was 8/1/2 months and ready to get it over with!

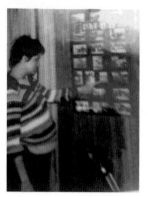 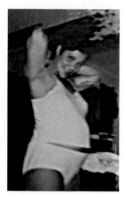

But I know better now that beauty comes from the inside. A person can be stunning, but if he or she is negative, which attracts negative energy and bias, then that person is ugly. How you choose to see reality determines your attitude in life, your success, your health, and your beauty.

Keep Laughing

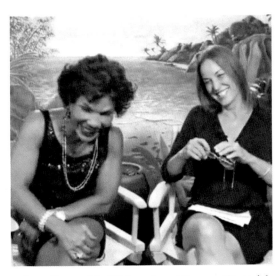

Josefina with TV co-host Laura Guttridge

I love to laugh. I think it's because I find joy in whatever I do.

My friend Cynthia, who is quite witty, makes ordinary events funny. It doesn't take much to get me laughing at her off the cuff remarks. One day we were at the gym, and as always, having a blast. The manager came and asked, "Would you mind not laughing. People are complaining that we're too happy." Lol

We assume that everyone wants to laugh, but maybe they never heard that sound in their family or they even discouraged it. Sad. If it's a question of how much to laugh, go all out. I laugh deeply from my belly, powerful and joyful. That has caused me some criticism; I am too happy for some people it seems.

Make laughing a part of your life every day. Like any habit you can make it happen. Develop a sense of humor. Find something funny or crazy you did, or something you heard during the day, and reflect on it unto you smile, or even laugh out loud. Would it be so bad if people pointed you out, saying, there she goes again, laughing to herself?

19

Laughter is happy therapy

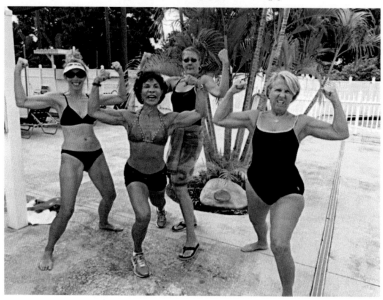

Don't forgot to have a good time

Laughter helps you to relax. It dissolves tension and reduces stress. Laughing decreases the secretion of the three major stress hormones: adrenaline, cortisol, norepinephrine. Your lymphatic and immune systems get a boost. I don't know if my systems enjoy laughter as much as I do, but it does give them the oomph to keep me healthy.

The scriptures speak of a happy heart as a medicine. If God says it and science confirms it, that's enough for me; let's keep on laughing!

Laughter:

- reduces pain—Laughter lessens pain when I train. It takes my mind off my muscles and puts it onto my belly. Of course, I am not encouraging you to lose focus.
- burns calories—A study showed that you burn 40 calories when you laugh for 15 minutes. That's a few pounds a year. Not bad for being happy.
- improves your mood—When you laugh, your brain releases endorphins, interferon-gamma (IFN), and serotonin. These are nature's feel-good chemicals that uplift your mood.

- infects others. When you are happy, so are those around you. But so also is negativity. Happy people gladden your heart; depressed people sadden it. Share your happiness and avoid the contagion of unhappy people.
- helps you get along with others—Laughing together create closeness, and a sense of trust, and builds co-operation. People are more willing to tell you things. Others want to be around you. And when there are problems (and there always are), it's easier to resolve them because people like and trust you.
- changes how you see things—You see things differently when you laugh. I ask myself, *What is the worst thing that can happen? Make a fool out of myself?* Not so bad in the scheme of things. It gives me a chance to laugh at myself, which keeps me humble. And it may make others happy, but in a good way, not laughing at me but with me.

I remember a situation in Washington, DC. I was at a social event hosted by Georgetown University. I had been studying there for only a few months and my English was limited. They were congratulating someone, and I translated the word "congratulation" into Spanish in my mind, extended my hand, and said to the person, "*Felicitacion jaja.*" To this day I still laugh at myself. *Jaja.*

Laughter makes you more secure, confident, and resilient. Life becomes tasty. Take a bite; delicious!

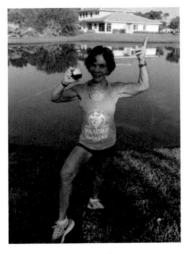

Keep Listening

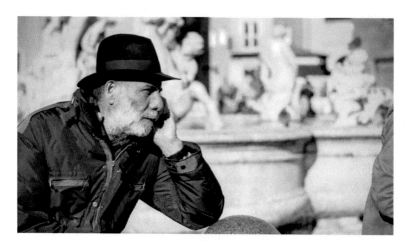

"Talk to someone about themselves and they'll listen for hours." That's the truth. I feel strongly about this quote by Dale Carnegie. We have lost the quality of attentive and active listening—being a great listener. Even with those closest to us, our attention span is small. Imagine how it is with strangers. I have accepted the fact that some people only want to be heard. So I let them talk. I have found that with these people it's better to listen than trying to share what's going on with me.

I have developed the skill of listening and being in the moment. It wasn't always this way. This happened to me all the time: someone would be talking to me and I remained engrossed about what I would say and not really listening. So now I wait and don't figure out what I'm going to say. Also, I take time before I decide to answer because many people don't really care about what you have to say. But when I really want someone to hear me—and they are not—I go straight to God and ask him to make it happen.

I find that it helps a person by just listening well. As people, talk they find a solution to the situation they are sharing with me. They just need a sounding board. Haven't you had that experience?

I talk at a different level of consciousness when I talk to God each morning during my daily ritual. He is the best listener; he hears what I have to say and then he answers me.

How do I know that?

One morning I was walking and jogging while crying and asking God for guidance. I was feeling lost and confused. I said to him, *Please, give me a sign that you are listing.*

My inner voice prompted me to go and take a sip of water in an area that I had never gone to for my water break. Although it is a private club and not open to the public, I still obeyed. I saw a water fountain on the deck. I walked toward it, and right in the center of the wooden planking was a turquoise ring. I bent down, picked it up, and put it on—it fit perfectly. My inner voice said, *It's my answer to your prayer.* Since then that ring represents my wedding to God. It is my true wedding ring.

I published on my YouTube channel an amazing story how one of my social media friends sent me a necklace that matches my ring beautifully. She never met me in person and had not seen my ring. And it was the first time I told this story so she could not have known about it. It's so encouraging to see God's confirmation of my relationship with him.

Here's a Facebook post I came across that sums it up nicely:

> This year, I'm going to concentrate on keeping my mouth shut and listening to you and others I encounter. It will be hard for me since all of you who actually know me personally, know that I love to talk and have lots of stories of my own. But, I'm going to work hard at using my ears and my mouth in the proportion I was born with. EVERYBODY HAS A STORY! I want to learn all the stories I can.[1]

Keep reminding yourself that it's ok just to listen. Learn to be a great listener.

---

[1] Helvey, Ed. Facebook. (January 1, 2018). What Will YOU Do With 2018? *Living Free Project.*
https://www.facebook.com/groups/529862534030273/permalink/563139 937369199/

Keep Loving

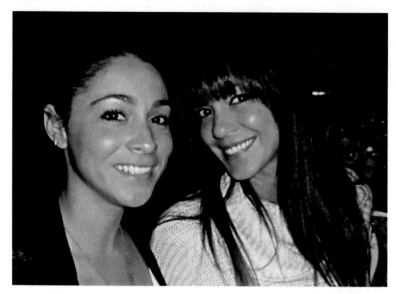

Love can't do its magical work if the busyness of life has you on a treadmill. Slow down. Don't be in a hurry. This way you'll be able to feel if someone could use a kind word or an encouraging smile.

Be a charming listener and others will feel at ease. They'll gladly talk with you about concerns on their minds and aches in their hearts. Your presence will comfort them because of your sincere interest in their well-being. They'll leave your presence better able to solve their problems. All because you slowed down as you passed by and listened. There is a saying I like: *Love makes the world go around.* Love is the essence of life. But how do we make it practical in everyday living?

To begin with, recognize where love comes from—God. Why is this important? There are three realms of reality: the material world (which includes our physical bodies), our minds (thoughts and feelings), and spirit (from which come our values—things like forgiveness, patience, and compassion). Developing a relationship with the source of love, our Father in heaven, enables love to flow into us. It's like energy in this sense. It's powerful as it charges us and energizes others as we let it flow through our vessels.

Before we can love another, we must first love ourselves. This sounds very nice and all, but how do you do it? That is where knowing God in a personal, very real way comes in. We are infants and children in this beginning of our eternal career. And don't we youngsters need our Father's comforting embrace, as he makes our boo-boos better?

For me, he encourages my efforts, tells me I am his own, assures me that what I consider shortcomings are merely baby steps in learning to walk in the way to eternity. I feel better about myself. I know I'm doing my best and my Father thinks so too. The result? I love myself. It's what self-respect is really about.

The next step to keep loving is to let love flow through you to others as mentioned earlier. This includes the values noted above: forgiveness, patience, compassion. But there are many more ways to let love flow through you by being:

loyal	genuine
truthful	sincere
sympathetic	noble
long-suffering	trusting
generous	honest
honorable	joyful
strong	righteous
gracious	friendly
cheerful	good

Seriously reflect on each value. How much is it your life? How often do you live it? It is through values like these that you show yourself loving.

Love in its essence is the desire to do good to others. So give a helping hand when you can. People will love you for it.

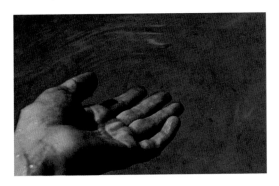

Keep Working on yourself

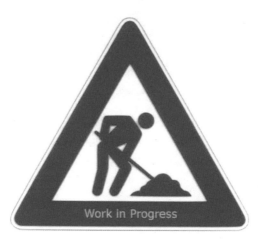

Work in Progress

Is this you? Are you really progressing?

Work has a bad rap. So does change. But they're not deserved. Think of work as progress, and change as growth. Work is not meant to be drudgery. If it seems so, there is a solution—the challenge of change. You have a decision about where to put your energy. I'm talking about your choice to age gracefully with strength and dignity. Or else agree with the naysayers who tell you to expect a withered and decrepit old age.

You have a choice to make. Will you work on yourself? I know, I know; I hear it often enough. *There's so much going on in my life, how can I possibly make working on myself a full time job, my central activity?* But what is the alternative? Give up? Surrender your well-being to doctors? Who knows your body better than you? It requires faith in your vision, commitment to do what it takes, investment of time, and the risk of setbacks.

Remarkable progress is being made in understanding how we age and how we can control it. You can benefit by aligning yourself with the body's innate process of restoration. Be open to seeing yourself, renewing your body continually. And when you do, you will age successfully.

But it's first needed to create a proactive mindset—not passive, not resistant to change. Change makes life an adventure. Embrace it, take charge, reach out, and make it happen. The result: the new you. But it does take commitment to:

- accept a new set of beliefs,

26

- mentally energize yourself every day,
- refuse the social pressure that you will age poorly.

In other words, take 100% charge of your health! I am not saying it is easy but I am saying it is possible. You need to believe, you need to be willing to give yourself a chance, you need to go it alone instead of going along to get along with all those who see aging as negative.

I have found it essential each day—that means *every* day—to work on my career of ageing well. I refuse to entertain thoughts of retirement from life. Doing this ensures that I am progressing in my life's purpose. It has been my calling from an early age to teach. Well, I am still teaching, still working, but in a different area of life. I stay engaged with life, I keep learning, I continue to thrive.

We are learning throughout our lives. It's how we're programmed: to keep working, finding, and reaching new levels of ourselves. We retain the capacity to change and learn, and it gets easier with the wisdom of experience as we grow older (now there's a benefit youth doesn't have yet).

The key to attain these new levels, the new you, is to rid yourself of anything that says you can't. Don't buy into the fallacy that you can't teach an old dog new tricks.

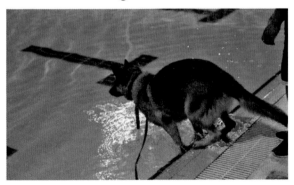

Keep reinventing yourself. You will find renewed purpose, and with it the energy that it brings. You need to feel fruitful, that your life has meaning. You need to have a reason why you're here; otherwise, give up, die, and go home. So what is your purpose? Let your unique personality show forth the beauty of your soul. Express it as loving service to all who come your way. What's deep within shines forth revealing the new you. You'll find the luminosity of your inner being attracts those would like the same.

27

Then you have the wonderful opportunity and satisfaction to share your life.

How to reinvent yourself

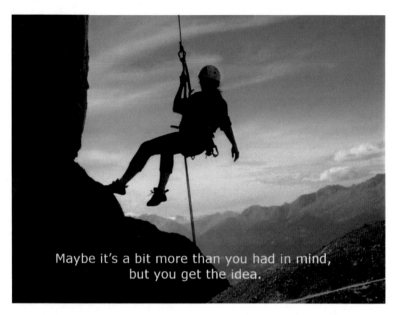

Maybe it's a bit more than you had in mind, but you get the idea.

A word about retirement. One source of the word is from the French *tirer* which means *to draw*. Retirement is an opportunity to *withdraw* from what you have been doing and *redraw* the canvas of your life. And you don't have to be a Rembrandt to be a co-creator of your life. There's artistry in that, wouldn't you say?

You may be open to learn something but don't have a clue how to go about it. If the desire is genuine and reflects who you really are, you will be led into it. It happened to me with bodybuilding. I had never heard about it, much less women competing. But I dared to put in the time, energy, discipline, personal commitment, and dedication to develop into an outstanding bodybuilder.

People sometimes get into what I call dissonance. It could be physical, mental, or emotional. It permeates their lives. They want to change but the energy of their beliefs stop them. There's a disconnect between what they believe and the new reality they want to embrace.

So how do you overcome dissonance? Beliefs carry energy. Each experience—physical, mental, emotional, even spiritual—is based on those energies. And most negative beliefs lodge in us as

28

children. Healing begins by recognizing each thought or feeling that makes you feel bad. Here's how one woman described it (slightly edited):

Energy within me was not freely flowing. My mind activity increased, my breathing became shallower, and there was tension and tiredness. I hadn't paid attention and failed to catch the rising dissonance the moment it began to form.[2]

After recognizing the negative thoughts and feelings, and then refusing to dwell on them, she simply released and let them go their way. Here is how she describes the moment of release when she realized what caused her to be uneasy.

I was looking at mere mental programming and nothing more or less than that. Something I was verbally fed with and it became my belief. Simple as that. I felt a release within my system, and the energy began to flow again in a matter of seconds. My tiredness dissipated immediately and clarity returned.

There's much written on how to go about it. And that takes work. So keep working.

In summary, with gladness take on the work of progressing each day toward health and well-being. It is never too late to learn new things. Keep challenging yourself. Onward and upward!

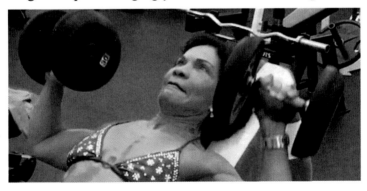

---

[2] Mayers, Christine. (2014). Moving Into Energetic Simplicity: How To Release Physical, Mental And Emotional Dissonance On The Level Of Energy. http://www.thenewempath.com/blog/answers-are-simple-the-mind-gets-lost-in-details

Keep the Mind Working Well

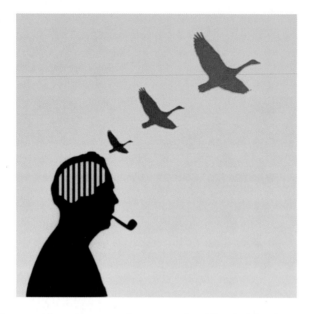

It is imperative that you become familiar with the magnificent endowment called mind. Why? Because everything begins with a thought—at least on a conscious level. Our thoughts (and this includes feelings, the thoughts of our emotions) reflect how we perceive the world; they become our reality. Meaningful and lasting change requires the consent of your mind.

Fundamental to taking control of your mind is your mental attitude. Embrace each negative thought and feeling as an insight that allows you to move beyond them. It's not so much introspection; that can draw you into an unproductive and time consuming revisit of hurt. Rather, it's a quick reflection of where the thought or feeling came from. And then let it go; release it; it no longer has a place in your life. If they are deeply embedded, they will arise again, so don't be dismayed. Just keep releasing them. And don't feel bad at yourself. God loves you and is watching and encouraging you as the loving divine Father that he is.

It is when you have become aware of your thoughts and feelings that you learn what is going on in your mind. You gain insight into why you are thinking and feeling these things. Then you can use your conscious mind in each situation to make the best of who you are. The most effective way to do this is by making a choice for the highest good for the most people for the longest time. Everything depends on this high spirit connection.

Reprogram your mind

There are three parts of the mind: conscious, subconscious, and superconscious. The conscious mind acts as the doorway to the subconscious. The job of the subconscious mind is to record whatever you are thinking and saying. Like a tape recorder it doesn't have a clue if what you are saying is truth or error. Whatever you are thinking imprints on your subconscious, so be extremely careful of your thoughts; don't indulge the bad ones!

It hurts you when you have trained your subconscious mind to believe: *I am too old; I'll never get my health back*; *this is the way things are, just live with it*. You can see how this damages your health. Fortunately, merely having the thought a few times will not harm you. Consistent repetition is what imprints it on your subconscious.

Mind programming works to our benefit as well. It is how you change from the negative to the positive, a person of dense and dark energies to one of higher vibrations of love and light. It is up to you to change the old negative programming and retrain your mind. Through your mind you create your own prophecy, and by its programming its fulfillment. Think of your subconscious as an airplane on automatic pilot. Once you, the captain of your destiny, set the course, that's where you will go—unless you decide with determined consciousness to change the course. Or think of the mind as a car. Your conscious mind is the driver; the subconscious powers the car. You, the driver, must learn to control and direct its power.

How sad that negative programming is imprinted during our earliest years. Parents sometimes belt their children with verbal two-by-fours until the child believes he or she is useless, stupid, and won't amount to anything; and on it goes.

In addition, our nature has taken in the emotional disruptors of our culture: fear, anger, greed, hatred, bigotry, violence, and lies. People lack the inner wellspring of love and solace that corrects and soothes these inner disturbances. They succumb to deep states of fear, afraid to recognize the pervasive error of their cultural and religious beliefs. Unstable emotions rise to the surface as emotional immaturity is unable to cope with them, thus allowing them to run rampant and cause fear and anxiety, a reason for the current epidemic of depression.

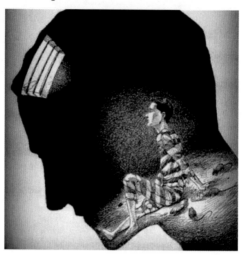

No wonder it is so difficult for people to change. You must make a conscious choice to turn your life around. Have a mental picture of the direction you want to go, and do what it takes to get there.

But most of us are on automatic pilot. Our subconscious rules. You can see it happening in your daily routine. You get up in the morning, brush your teeth, drive your car or ride a bike, all without much thought; you do it automatically! Ever been driving and ten minutes later realize that you had no idea you were driving? Your mind took off without you.

Why do you think and feel things without conscious awareness? Because once you train yourself, or your parents train you, you no longer need to think consciously about it. The subconscious mind doesn't argue with you, it just does whatever it has been programmed to do, whether it is good for you or not.

Does any of the following self-talk ring a bell as it reinforces a false image of who you are?

- I have no control about my weight.
- My thyroid is a mess.
- I always get the rotten end of the deal.
- Life is a bitch. It's not worth trying. I already know what will happen.

Like they say in the computer world: garbage in, garbage out. Now you can see how important is to know how your biological computer works. It does not think, reason, or deliberate, but it can be reprogrammed—thank God for that!

The creative mind

When you have an issue, a problem, and want to do something but don't know how, the creative mind solves the problem for you. *Sleep on it.* A saying well founded on answers coming to you during the night seasons so you awake knowing what to do. We've all had the experience.

Here's how it works. The reservoir of thoughts, ideas, and experiences in the subconscious undergo a process of association by which new neural connections are made and the resultant thoughts rise to the conscious mind upon waking. Likewise, ideals and meanings and values descend from the superconscious into the conscious mind and you're inspired to do things in a higher way.

It's not important to know how it all works, but that it does. So you when get that inspiration, that illumination, that Aha! moment, be confident in it being right. Recognize it's real and act on it.

The mind is picture oriented

I learned that the mind is picture oriented when very young. I pictured what I wanted. As I focused on and kept the picture before me it became vivid and eventually indelible. When visualizing, you don't see words, you see pictures. If I say to you "apple" or "one hundred dollars," you don't see the *word* "apple" or the words "one hundred dollars"; you see the pictures of an apple and a $100 bill.

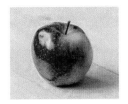 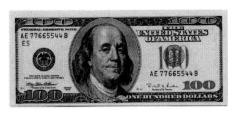

There comes a moment when your visualization, the picture you hold in your mind, grows stronger than your present reality. POW! That's when your determination comes into play. You control moving toward the new reality created in your mind by

33

visualizing the new you, your new reality. This is how to make lasting and meaningful change, when the new picture of reality becomes your life.

Remember that your perceptions create your reality. The new picture becomes reality through continual and constant visualization. The concept behind the picture integrates into the neural structure of your brain. Your life situation is a product of your perceptions and your creative subconscious process. Your creative subconscious works to make sure that the picture you hold on the inside (your vision) matches what you see on the outside (your reality). Thus a new reality comes into being. Hallelujah!

The two pictures must match. If not, then you have cognitive dissonance, meaning you hold two conflicting thoughts—inner turmoil. The one that wins is the one you believe in the strongest. So be exceedingly careful what pictures you hold in your mind.

My change began by seeing myself in my next station in life, a new world and a new reality. That's why when people would tell me, "You won't make it" because of my current situation, I would ignore *their* picture of my future. Instead it caused me to focus and strengthen *my* picture of my new reality. Not just once, but over and over until my mental picture strengthened, daily becoming more powerful. The seeming unending assault on what I foresaw for myself energized me. I could taste my future! POW!

In my first book, *Vibrant at Any Age,* I explain step by step how to make your new vision real.

Keep Meditating

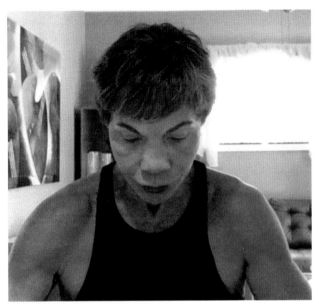

Meditation is a state of consciousness. Your physical body needs a balanced, disciplined mind. Meditating each day provides that discipline, allowing your mind to be clear, peaceful, cool and collected. Meditation means to me inner peace.

Here is how I meditate and some of its benefits:

- I don't have to sit in a particular way to meditate. I discovered that I can meditate anytime and anywhere. One of my favorite is what I call "walking meditation." I walk every morning three miles during which I commune with God.
- I talk to God literally. Most of the time I thank him for how wonderful he is to me. Other times I tell him how I am feeling about problems. At other times I sing. But always am I mindful of the beauty, sounds, and smells of creation.
- After I walk three miles, I jog back another three and my meditation is usually prayer. I feel out for the needs of others and ask God to make them receptive to his will for them. Also that they feel his love and watch care.
- Meditation allows me to stay in the present moment; the past and future doesn't exist, only the here and now.

- Meditation is nutrition for my spirit, and at the same time it provides me with physical benefits. One of them is that I feel rested and peaceful.
- Meditation reduces my level of stress. I find myself spending less time anxious about life's difficulties or others people's dramas.
- My muscles relax instead of being tense and tight.
- It rejuvenates me. It diminishes the lines in my face giving me the look of Botox or some kind of filler, but less expensive and more rewarding.
- Meditation frees me from fear about life and death. It does the opposite, instilling a sense of freedom.
- It gives me dynamic energy to be cheerful; I feel powerful with boundless energy.

You can achieve these benefits and more by including meditation as a part of your daily routine.

Entering into meditation

- Set up a special area in your home to meditate. I have several areas conducive to meditation. Let it be quiet and without distractions. Make it a sacred place. Have pictures of God, create an altar. I usually have fresh flowers in my home which helps. Be creative in setting the scene to meditate.
- You can use scents from candles and incense to set the mood to meet your best self.
- Wear comfortable clothes.
- Take a yoga class. It is good training for meditation.
- Repeat a mantra or affirmation to enter into quietness. Or you can look at the ocean or choose any element that you love, and that will help you to develop focus and concentration. During my walking meditation in the morning I focus on the beauty around me in all its magnitude and magnificence.
- If you choose to meditate in the evening, then develop a ritual that will prepare you for it. Like taking a shower, relaxing your body, clearing your mind. Let everything go that happened during your day.

More thoughts on meditation.

Meditation is not the eastern guru sitting cross-legged staring off into space. What it means is deep reflection. After quieting your mind you are able to commune with your innermost being—God within. I mean that literally because a spirit fragment of the Infinite God lives within each of our minds and is dedicated to our well-being.

Ideally, put aside time each day and consciously invite God to commune with you. Make it the best time of your day; always give God your best. During your time alone in the garden of your soul speak with your Father in heaven. Ask him questions and discuss challenges for which you would like his counsel. Above all, feel the love of your real Father as he comforts you. Let him tell you how worthy and valuable you are, how he has always loved, wanted, and cherished you.

> You only have to quiet your mind…and learn to listen from the inside in order to perceive the rightful course of action to undertake.[3]

It is during this time of stillness that errant thoughts and feelings arise to distract you. Develop the discipline of determined effort to recognize and release these distracting thoughts and feelings until stillness becomes your life. You will learn that most of what you think and how you react originate outside of you, from your parents, from the culture, from what you think is expected of you, from so-called conscience that is not really you.

There will come a time when you no longer battle things from without. You will enjoy your time alone with God. Should thoughts or feelings arise to disturb your peace, it is good practice to reflect on your heavenly Father, that he loves you and accepts you just as you are. He has planned your future and has charted the way through it. You have but to cooperate, which is what you are doing by mastering your mind.

You can train your mind. The practice of mind-mastery is called *mindfulness*. However, few people do so because the mind is barely understood; it seems to have a "mind of its own." But it can be brought into submission to your ideals and spiritual values.

---

[3] D'Ingillo, Donna. (2017). Divine Mother, Divine Father: Teachings on Inspired Living from Our Heavenly Parents. San Rafael, CA: Origin Press. p.46.

That's when you feel good about yourself, standing tall in the radiance of your inner beauty—self-respect.

However, it is important not to confuse mindfulness with reflective meditation, which is communion with God Within. Mindfulness is a tool to help you achieve loving and friendly conversation with God, he who is behind the scenes, living in your superconscious mind from whence he diligently attempts to impart his guidance. The superconscious links you to the portal of the cosmic realm from whence you receive the real meanings of things and the true values to live by. Meditation, or deep reflection, opens the door to the super-human realm of your mind.

As you master your mind and grow in your relationship with God, others feel the energies of your thoughts and emotions emanating from you. You are sharing your life in service to their welfare. Love in action; how it should be.

The Seven Steps of Stillness

(copyright Center for Christ Consciousness
www.ctrforchristcon.org/the-stillness.html)

It helps to have structure in learning to meditate or enter into stillness. The Center for Christ Consciousness has graciously allowed these proven steps to be reprinted. They are intended to help you connect with your Inner Spirit, to train your mind to become more Father centered and directed.

STEP 1: Physical Relaxation

Being physically relaxed is very important so you can remain in the stillness undisturbed by discomfort. Choose a comfortable position whether sitting or reclining that will keep you awake and aware. Now, take several deep breaths and release them slowly. Let your body thoroughly unwind. Close your eyes and let yourself thoroughly relax.

STEP 2: Mental Stillness

The mind is naturally active – thoughts, worries, plans, fears and anxieties can all come rushing in. Tell your mind to "be still!" Pick a centering point: repeat a mantra, listen to instrumental music, visualize a pleasant scene to refocus your thoughts when your mind begins to wander. If you find other thoughts come into your mind, simply re-focus on your centering point. Then, when you feel relaxed and at peace, direct your thoughts to opening to the relationship you share with your Inner Spirit and begin:

STEP 3: Talk to God

Within your being is the best friend, wisest counselor, and most loving parent you will ever know. Share with your internal source what is on your mind and in your heart. Your Inner Spirit is your direct connection to God—your Divine Source, who knows you intimately and accepts you just the way you are. In the same manner as you would share your day with a spouse or a close companion, share it with God. You do the talking; God is doing the listening.

STEP 4: Ask for Help

This is your time to ask for help, which could also be called prayer. From the previous step, you may ascertain where and what kind of spiritual help you need from your Spirit Parent. Remember, there is always a solution; everything is resolvable with God's help. If you do not know what to ask for, ask your Inner Spirit, "What do I need now to grow spiritually?" Also, spend a few moments praying for others – you say the prayer for them that they cannot say for themselves.

STEP 5: Give Thanks

This is the step to simply give thanks and appreciation for everything good in life that has been given as a gift. Offer your appreciation and praise to the Divine Source of everything true, beautiful, and good. What do you have to be thankful for? Everything! Life, love, family, friends, health. Recognize the Divine Hand in your life and simply acknowledge Spirit's contribution.

STEP 6: Silent Listening

Now is the time to listen within—What does your Inner Voice wish to say to you? Return to your centering point, tune your listening within and wait. You may not hear a booming voice telling you what to do, but you may begin to perceive that God is trying to talk to you from afar; the message may only be subtly and faintly discerned. You may even think you haven't received anything at this time. But later, tomorrow, or in a few days suddenly an answer will flash into your mind, or someone may say the words you need to hear, or you might find them in a book. It takes a while sometimes for the Spirit Within to pierce through the static layers of consciousness. But rest assured, your Inner Voice will indeed respond.

STEP 7: The Embrace

Receive the love and guidance God has for you. By opening your heart and mind from the previous steps, it is now your time to just relax and receive. Envision and sense yourself in the most beautiful and loving situation you have ever experienced, and ask for Spirit to amplify that feeling in you. You will become refreshed and renewed from within. Your Divine Source is feeding you internally; this is your soul's nourishment. The more you experience LOVE, the more you accumulate the desire to be in that state. And the more God's LOVE and wisdom radiates within you, the more you take into the outer world. Life begins to unfold in faith and joy!

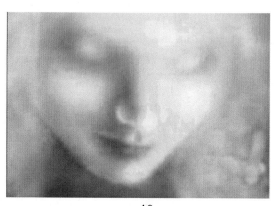

Keep Serving

The high destiny of the individual is to serve rather than to rule.
(Albert Einstein)

Everyone talks about love. But that's all it is, talk, until you do something about it. That's what service is all about. You care enough for others that when someone comes your way who can use your help, you're right there reaching out with a helping hand.

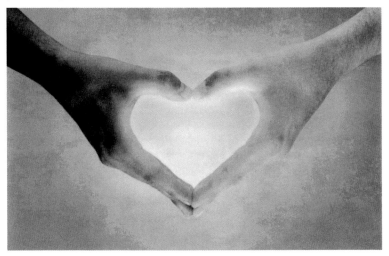

I'm always talking about becoming all you can be. Why is that? Because you can't help someone else until you have helped yourself. To do your part, you must first become whole yourself. That's why I talk about eliminating the negative and accentuating the positive, about reinventing yourself, moving on to new challenges and difficulties that bring forth your potential and make it actual.

The natural state of the human body is health and vitality. It comes from stepping out of the old belief system that retirement is to sit on a rocking chair and wait to die.

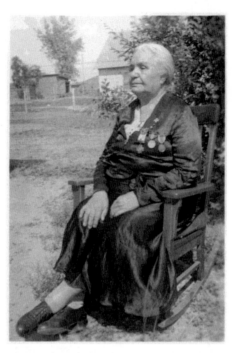

Well, guess what. If you do that you will die! Studies show that it's not healthy to give up living fully because of the number of years on your clock or it's the way things are supposed to be.

When we engage life and grasp the wonderful opportunities it presents, we become a better person and a real motivator and encourager to others. When we focus our life on service, whatever our capacity to do so, we are rewarded with a stronger sense of purpose and meaning, and that leads to better mental and physical well-being.

My question to you: *Why not continue discovering your talents? Why not challenge yourself instead of sitting on that old rocking chair?*

I am not talking about just getting out of the house and doing things to stay occupied and pass the time so you're not bored. I am talking about activities that begin a new career for you, a new challenge, something different, something that gets you excited to be alive! Something that gives you more meaning and greater power to do good. I am talking about a new you, so when you look at yourself in the mirror you say, oh my God! I never knew I could be so awesome.

It helps to have a mentor or a coach who knows the goals you are after and works with you to develop new skills to reach them.

As an example, I needed a coach for bodybuilding. I hadn't a clue what bodybuilding was or how to train. Forget about competing, it was not even a thought in my mind. That's exactly what I told Steve Pfeaster, my coach and mentor in the sport of bodybuilding. In six months he took me to my first competition where I successfully began my new adventure of personal development and reinventing myself.

You can't stand still and go places. It requires faith that you are not alone in your quest to become a whole, unified, loving human being. It requires courage to try something new. It requires wisdom to know how to go about it.

I've learned that when I'm supposed to start up a new path that I get help. We have talents that are ready to be developed at certain times in our lives; for me it has been every ten years. For example, I couldn't be a writer in my twenties, forties, or even my fifties and sixties. Why? Because I didn't have the life experience needed. But finally I did and here's how it came about.

I was feeling stuck when I was ready to move to south Florida, that I wasn't pursuing my next goal to be a writer. Everyone would ask, *Have you written a book?* Yes, I wanted to but I had no idea how to start. Then one day, POW! I met my coach and mentor, Richard Rosen, who has guided me every step of the way. Richard is a prolific writer. He has written many books about spirituality. Our personalities complement each other. That has been the main reason for the success of my books.

Beneath the mantle of my life is the bedrock of service, uplifting others as others have lifted me up. It's a two-way street. If you want to achieve your goals, become centered in living for others, adding value to their lives. Becoming all you are purposed to be increases your capacity to help others become all they are purposed to be. The end result? Heaven on earth.

Why is this? Each of us is endowed with a personality from our heavenly Father. You are designed to serve an eternal purpose, to take your rightful place in our cosmic family and there do your part. In the same way we each have a role to play here. Only your unique personality with its attributes can do its part to progress society. Only you, by caring for others in a way that only you can, enables them to rise up to the challenges of life and become better. We're all in this together and we each do our part by loving service as occasion allows.

43

Here is something else about service. It's so rewarding when you help someone. There's a feeling that goes to your soul. It's like heaven saying, *I'm proud of you my child*. It makes life worthwhile. It makes you want to do more.

And this is how the world gets better. As more people show their love by helping others, society advances and civilization progresses. We each have our part. It begins by becoming all you are purposed to be, and doing the same for others. It's a great journey. *Vaya con Dios!*

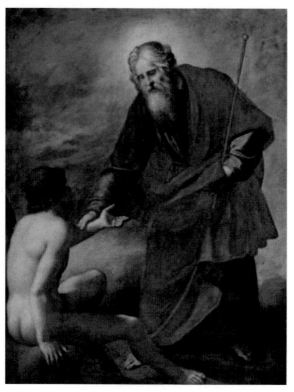

Keep Being a Whole Person

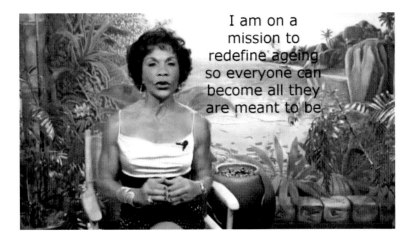

Most people focus on the physical part of themselves, their bodies. It's understandable, it being material and all too often giving you a pain you can't ignore. Nonetheless, neglect not the whole you: spiritual, mental, emotional, and physical—and if possible, in this order. You become a unified personality when you take care of your spirit, mind, and body. Your emotions are balanced and in harmony with your thoughts. You achieve emotional and intellectual maturity as well as moral integrity.

Here's the most important thing you can do to grow the better you. *Each* day still your mind, link up to the Spirit Within, and glean the handfuls of purpose that enrich your life. Everything else follows and is secondary.

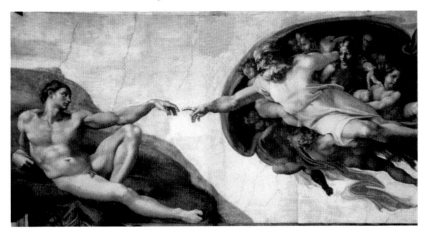

Harmonize the energies of your body, mind, and spirit to become a person of poise. For the body it means avoiding the poisons of chemicalized processed food and a toxic environment. For the mind it means identifying poisonous thoughts and harmful feelings and releasing them. For the spirit it means letting go the dark energies of feeling unloved and embracing a relationship with God Within, hearing from and following his loving guidance.

Be prepared. A dominating poison in your life does not leave easily. It takes intelligent effort, and equally—or perhaps more important—perseverance. Don't give up. Over time you begin to see the results of your effort by recognizing motives that led you into the behaviors you are seeking to change. As a corollary, you will become more confident in who you are—self-respect.

Keep Learning what God Says about Health and Ageing

I know the Bible isn't an anchor to the soul for some as it is for me. So I will explain the verses that are valuable to my life, hoping you will find meaning in them as well.

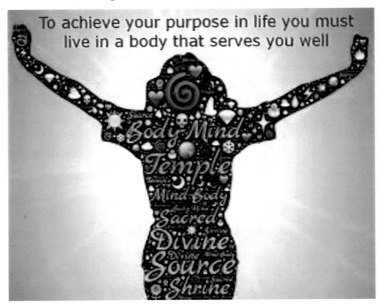

To reach a goal in life we must stand on beliefs that support us. When it comes to slowing down the ageing process, I stand on God's word, what he says about it. Deeply reflecting on Truth, whatever its source, infuses you with understanding, energy, and direction. For me, the scriptures are the rock on which I stand. Here are some that work for me.

> Do you not know that your body is a temple of the Holy Spirit within you, whom you have from God? You are not your own, for you were bought with a price. So glorify God in your body. (1 Corinthians 6:19,20)

My interpretation of this beautiful scripture is that my body is the house of the Holy Spirit. Because this is so, why would I make a mess of the dwelling place where the holy part of me lives? Because my body is on loan from the Spirit that he might live through me, it belongs to her and not me. I am its caretaker and am responsibility to be a good one. I am accountable to nurture and protect my tabernacle of flesh so when it is time to move on to my heavenly home, I will leave it in the best possible condition. It's like moving out of a rental property; you leave it as good or *better* than when you moved in.

And so it is with your temple of the living God who lives within you. Prepare your body and mind to be the most wholesome and beautiful you can, that it may house a soul of nobility. Then shall people take note that you walk with God.

So, whether you eat or drink, or whatever you do, do all to the glory of God. (I Corinthians 10:31)

When you eat something, be mindful if God approves. Wholesome food makes it easier to hear from your Spirit.

For while bodily training is of some value, godliness is of value in every way, as it holds promise for the present life and also for the life to come. (1 Timothy 4:8)

Balance the time and effort you put into your physical body. Do not neglect the morals of high living and the values of spiritual communion in your effort to optimize your body.

A joyful heart is good medicine, but a crushed spirit dries up the bones. (Proverbs 17:22)

God wants you happy. Gladness of spirit makes for a healthy heart and body. Therefore, whenever you find yourself sad, confused, or lonely, get in touch with God who lives within and have a heart-to-heart talk.

And God said, "Behold, I have given you every plant yielding seed that is on the face of all the earth, and every tree with seed in its fruit. You shall have them for food. (Genesis 1:29)

Eat what God has made; avoid chemicalized and adulterated man-made processed food.

For you were bought with a price. So glorify God in your body. (1 Corinthians 6:20)

Did you know that God is happy when you take care of your body? More than that, he can talk with you and work through you that much more effectively when you avoid and rid yourself of noxious food and environmental toxins.

I can do all things through him who strengthens me. (Philippians 4:13)

No matter what shape you're in, and how hard it seems to get your life back on track, your connection with God ensures you will get there. Think about it: is there anything too hard for God?

I appeal to you therefore, brothers, by the mercies of God, to present your bodies as a living sacrifice, holy and acceptable to God, which is your spiritual worship. (Romans 12:1)

You want to worship God? Begin with a body that's in good shape. You're doing it to please God, not to have everyone tell you how great you look.

Do not be conformed to this world, but be transformed by the renewal of your mind, that by testing you may discern what is the will of God, what is good and acceptable and perfect. (Romans 12:1-2)

Before your body can be healthy, your mind must be in the right place. And where's that? Your greatest desire is to know what God wants you to do, and then you do it. Good things will follow, as morning does the night, when you have a healthy relationship with God.

I praise you, for I am fearfully and wonderfully made. Wonderful are your works; my soul knows it very well. (Psalm 139:14)

Did you ever think how intricately and beautifully our bodies are put together? It's not by random events and happenstance, but by the divinely managed evolution of our physical systems. You are its caretaker.

Wine is a mocker, strong drink a brawler, and whoever is led astray by it is not wise. (Proverbs 20:1)

Clear instruction: whether it's alcohol, drugs, or an addiction of habit, discipline yourself. Remember, with God all things are possible.

Be not wise in your own eyes; fear the Lord, and turn away from evil. It will be healing to your flesh and refreshment to your bones. (Proverbs 3:7)

I reflected on scriptures that deal with bones when I was having issues with my hips; and it worked. Whenever I had a challenge in my life, I would choose the scriptures that pertained to it. I would stand upon them as the rock of my assurance that I am invincible, that I will resolve the situation. I would talk with God and call to mind the verses until the issue was resolved.

She dresses herself with strength and makes her arms strong. (Proverbs 31:17)

This verse resonates with me. I looked back on all the way God has led me, and I said to him, *Yes! You have strengthened me physically, mentally, and spiritually for the work you set before me.* What a confirmation of my purpose in life. POW!

Then Psalm 103 furthered my reflection, especially the last line.

Bless the Lord, O my soul, and all that is within me, bless his holy name!
Bless the Lord, O my soul, and forget not all his benefits, who forgives all your iniquity, who heals all your diseases, who redeems your life from the pit, who crowns you with steadfast love and mercy,
who satisfies you with good *so that your youth is renewed like the eagle's.*

The Scriptures I have shared with you epitomize being healthy, young, and vibrant at any age. It can be summarized in Isaiah 40:31.

But they who wait for the Lord shall renew their strength; they shall mount up with wings like eagles; they shall run and not be weary; they shall walk and not faint.

This is why I choose to believe my youth renews in strength like an eagle. It is why I stand on this belief. My faith charts a new course in unknown waters; it discovers a land of new opportunities to claim; it masters a new territory.

And so it is with each of us who link up with God. Life is never dull, but an adventure in which we together co-create the way

51

forward. How exciting to have God as your navigator! Hoist your mainsail and let the wind of Spirit move you.

* * *

Here is a question: Is having a well-turned body and a sound mind sufficient to be *vibrant at any age*? You're in the section about God's view of aging, so my answer is that God has made a *three* stranded cord of well-being that unifies the whole person: body-mind-spirit.

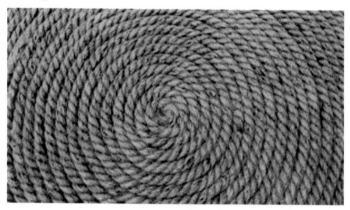

Applying science to optimize your health supports a mind capable of pursuing wisdom, the philosophy of life that guides you. But marshaling the facts of science and the philosophy that yields wisdom leads to the third domain of the whole person: spirit. This is where mind leaves off and the soul grows from insight into truth that is only spiritually perceived—truths of the heart, your innermost being.

So while building your body and satisfying your mind, neglect not the nourishment of your soul, which instructs from whence you come, why you are you are here, and where you are going. The result: a person of beauty, a mind of tranquility, and a soul of nobility.

How do you live each day? This message gives a wonderful perspective.

What you do with your day is, of course, up to you. You all have work to do to maintain your material existence. But what do you do each day to maintain your spiritual existence? This is up to you as well. Equally as important as your material needs are your spiritual needs. For example, how much love do you need each day to be fulfilled? How much peace, how much patience, how much tolerance, how much understanding of others? These are real needs, my child, and I ask you to look at each one more carefully. What will you do each day to meet your spiritual needs to your satisfaction?[4]

The optimization of your physical, mental, emotional, and spiritual states has a purpose beyond the pleasure of self-mastery. Life is about relationships, social relations with your fellows. You need to optimize them as much as the rest of you. Love, be compassionate, and uplift your brothers and sisters. It could be a smile, a word of encouragement, help with a task, work in a social service organization, or heart words that quicken the soul. And so your whole being comes full circle to enter in to the next life with a character of strength and a soul of nobility.

God centered posts

Be ever mindful of God as you take control of the aging process. Here are several posts from my social media.

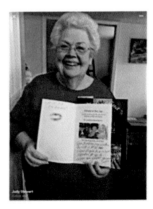

Now that you came into my life I can enjoy the rest of it! The Lord told me several years ago that I thought my life was over, but it is just beginning.

I believe that you are part of his plan for my life. Being connected to the Lord, like you are, got my attention. I can look back and see that all my life he has been in control, just like putting you in my path. Since God is my Father, that makes

---

[4] D'Ingillo, Donna. (2016). Divine Mother, Divine Father: Messages on Inspired Living from Our Heavenly Parents. Origin Press. (p.70).

us sisters, and I love you dearly. POW! B.D.

I read about you on MSN today. I was so inspired that I had to follow you. The article was like God speaking to me through you. Glad we have strong, positive people like you who break the norms and we can look up to. God bless. L.A.

Awesome Testimony! I feel so blessed that the Holy Spirit led me to your video messages. I am 40 years old and for the last year I have been struggling with my health and feeling hopeless and depressed, as though it's only going to get worst.

For the past two weeks I have been listening to your video messages and the Holy Spirit is rejuvenating my spirit. I listened to a message of yours today where you said, *As we age, we should be getting, stronger, soaring, powerful and overcoming.* A message that hit me to the core: God purposes for me to live a full life, getting better every day!

Thank you so much for allowing the Holy Spirit to use you to revive my spirit! V.M.

Everyday I look towards God for advice and encouragement no matter what I'm facing, good or bad. He is always my safe place and I know I can count on him ALWAYS. He is my main motivator.

After God I look for people like this amazing woman, and others like her, to pep me up and get me going every day. This lady has an amazing attitude. She loves God, life, people, and is strong. And, oh yeah, she's 71 years young! J.

God knew exactly what I needed to see and read today. I came across one of your videos a while ago. I did not come across it by mistake.

I am a 52 year old who just went back to school to get my nursing license. My age has made me a little self-conscious. I have always tried to work on a healthy body and eating, but sometimes I fall short. Since I have been in school I have really fallen short and can feel it.

I have been beating myself up about my age. Seeing this gives me the incentive to be proud that I am in nursing school. I know

now, after seeing your video how you started working out, there is still hope for this 52 year old. Thank you.

Well I guess my hunch was correct. That makes us sisters in Christ. I am beginning my journey to reach a goal I had even in high school but have not attempted until now (I am 52). I always had an interest in body building or a similar venture. Long story but your book is helping me move out of some negative areas into the positive. This path is a gift from God he has enlightened for me. L.

A prayer: I pray my Father that you give me the strength, discipline, commitment, courage, and the renewing of my mind to have this restoring power as this wonderful woman has in her life. We all have things that need to be changed for the better. Help me God restore my body to what it should be. And thank you for letting me come across this woman and her teachings to help me achieve what's best for me! K.C.

Whoever ever gets to be in your company will have such a high on life because you are a childlike spirited Christian—which we rarely see. Plus you have extreme discipline, which also is rare. Such a spectacular combination makes you a great inspiration and testimony to our perfect Lord and Savior. You truly glorify Him every time I see you—full of the JOY OF THE LORD! Thank you for sharing your life with us and being an exemplary sister.

P.S. You blessed me by talking to ME—PERSONALLY—and praying for me on YOUR LIVE VIDEO! You put the needs of a stranger before anything and got others to pray for me too. May God encourage you, my precious sister—abundantly—as you have done for me, just one li'l sheep—a little sad and lonely, but much less now! BLESS YOU JOSEPHINA!

Final thoughts

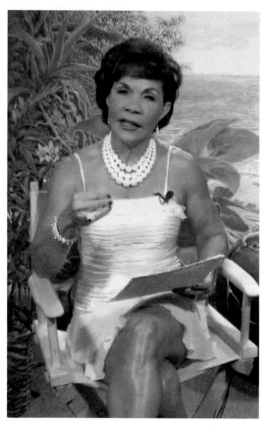

This poem by Ralph Waldo Emerson describes what a successful life is all about. I identify with it; perhaps you will too.

- To laugh often and much;
- to win respect of intelligent people and the affection of children;
- to earn the appreciation of honest critics and endure the betrayal of false friends;
- to appreciate beauty;
- to find the best in others;
- to leave the world a bit better whether by a healthy child, a garden patch, or a redeemed social condition;
- to know even one life has breathed easier because you have lived.
- *This is to have succeeded.*

Keep yourself encouraged

I received a request to be interviewed for a TV documentary to inspire people to think about their fitness regardless of age, using the interviewer's life as an illustration. Here is part her email that I hope inspires you to plan and preserve your health and fitness all the remaining years of your life.

I am working for the UK based TV company on a documentary celebrating the journey to old age. The program will push boundaries, show the unexpected and recognize honestly that at 60 years old, there is a generation still facing a third of their lives—life isn't over!

I hope to illustrate the inspiration I have gained from you to push myself as far as possible, to remain healthy and fit in my later years. I am grateful for the opportunity to develop a strong and healthy body which will surely keep illness at bay.

What she has begun so can you!

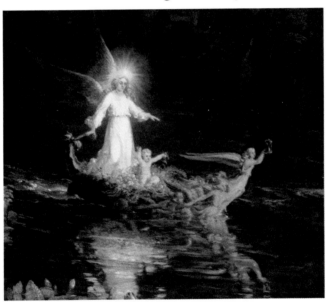

You are cared for and watched over

Onward, Upward, and Inward

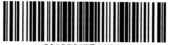

36135217R00040